Hearts or Hernias?

Audrey Goldhawk

An Authors OnLine Book

Copyright © A Goldhawk 2010

Cover design by Siobhan Smith ©

All rights reserved. No part of this publication may be reproduced, stored in a retrieval system, or transmitted in any form or by any means, electronic, mechanical, photocopy, recording or otherwise, without prior written permission of the copyright owner. Nor can it be circulated in any form of binding or cover other than that in which it is published and without similar condition including this condition being imposed on a subsequent purchaser.

British Library Cataloguing in Publication Data.
A catalogue record for this book is available from the British Library.

ISBN 978 0 7552 0628 5

Authors OnLine Ltd
19 The Cinques
Gamlingay, Sandy
Bedfordshire SG19 3NU
England

This book is also available in e-book format, details of which are available at www.authorsonline.co.uk

My grateful thanks to the following family and friends for their help and encouragement – Jane and Alan for the typing and arranging, Hilary and Tom, Judith and Andrew, Joyce, Barbara and Jim.

My dear friend, Beau, died shortly before this little book of memories had been completed.

A.G.

November 2010

A. G. Goldhawk

The copy of the postcard of West Herts Infirmary, Hemel Hempstead is from the collection at Hertfordshire Archives & Local Studies, County Hall, Hertford, SG13 8EJ.

- Starting Out 3
    - Early Days 4
    - Male Surgical Ward 6
    - Eye Ward 8
    - Night Duty and Babies 9
    - Days Off 11
    - Women's Medical Ward 15
    - Odd Jobs 16
    - Patient Care 18
    - Exams 20
- Illness Strikes 23
- Starting Again 35
    - Training Again 36
    - Maternity Ward 36
    - Christmas on the Wards 38
    - Men's Medical on Nights 40
    - Friends 42
    - Life and Death 44
    - Ups and Downs 45
    - The Theatre 47
    - Important Visitors 49
    - Strange Ops 51
    - Theatre Relief 52
    - Ward Rounds 54
    - Emergencies 56
    - Children's Ward – Kippers All Round 58
    - Strange Fruit 60
    - Social Work 60
    - Happy Time 63
    - Kitchens 65
    - Royalty 67
    - Wedding Rings 67
    - Rail Crash 69
    - Strains 70
- Final Exams 73
    - Testing Times 73
    - Orals 74
    - Results 75
    - Contract of Service 77

Nursing in the 1940s

Chapter One

Starting Out
Derby Royal Infirmary

A cold wet blustery March morning greeted me – what would this day bring for me?

It was the first day on my journey to become a State Registered Nurse.

The cold train did nothing to cheer me, after a long night of tossing and turning as my mind scurried back and forth in nervous anticipation. I longed to hide myself in a corner seat – but no! It was not to be – I was to stand or perch on my case in the corridor which seemed full with other weary travellers – mostly members of H.M. Forces. The three-hour journey to Derby eventually ended and I found myself walking along a rather dim and foreboding street which led to the large Victorian-looking building ahead – the huge iron gates had been removed for the 'war effort' and the imposing statue of Florence Nightingale before me dominated the whole scene. Those eyes seemed inescapable.

Early Days

At last, taking my courage in both hands, I walked through the massive doors and gingerly approached the desk in the reception area. I explained my mission and was directed to one of the hierarchy of the hospital in her cosy office. She greeted me kindly and for the sum of one shilling and three pence handed me a 'student nurse' badge. She wished me a happy and profitable three years. Then, taking my hand, she said, "Good luck, Nurse", my training had begun – did she really call me Nurse? The idea seemed quite amusing.

My next stop was the Nurses' Home, which was made up of two wings – one old and the other considerably newer.

Home Sister greeted me and sent a maid to show me to my room. It was situated in the older part of the building – too bad, I thought. I found a notice awaiting me – it was telling me to be in a certain room in the evening to meet the other girls who had arrived, and we had to present ourselves to the Junior Sister Tutor. We all looked pretty nervous as we were handed our uniform after much measuring and fitting! All articles of clothing were to have our surnames embroidered on them within a fairly limited time. Fortunately my surname was short, but it was hard luck on the girl with thirteen letters in her name.

Sister welcomed us now as a 'School' of twelve hopeful girls, but now, she continued, "You are young women in training for the next three years"– she trusted they would be happy and fruitful years! After speaking to the other 'young women', and realising that we all shared one common feeling – panic – I went to my room. There the case must be unpacked and various knick knacks placed around to give a slightly more homely feeling to the bare room.

The Nurses' Home was made up of several concrete corridors with bedrooms leading off on either side.

I was soon to find out the method of alarm in the morning. At just around 6.30 a.m. a maid walked down the corridor opening each door, accompanied by a very loud "Morning Nurse" and slamming of the door with all her might – I immediately knew that she had the most well developed arm muscles in the city. She left behind rooms of shaking creatures, ears wrapped in pillows, all trying to protect their pink shells from permanent damage.

Now it was School, beginning at 8.30 a.m., and lasting for three months with one day off each week.

Sister Tutor was a very attractive young lady and also a very kind, though strict, person, helping the School to bond well – a bond which has lasted with some friends for sixty-odd years.

School was an intense time of lectures, tests, practical work and learning to make beds with the all important hospital corner! Jimmy, the skeleton, had to put up with pokes and probes as we learned where organs were situated and the plastic model was riddled with pin pricks from our first attempts to give injections! And then there was the everlasting bandage practice!

At last we faced the examinations – written and oral. I had found the studying required during the three months very difficult. Coming from a small rural school, I had left at fourteen years of age – I was badly equipped for all the work my little grey cells were to encounter. Fortunately, there was one particular girl who had been favoured with a good education – it was Joyce who assisted me through the maze of study books, and our friendship still remains sixty odd years on.

Having passed the entrance examination, some of the School decided to celebrate – tomorrow we were going to our appointed ward and practical nursing would begin in earnest.

We were in high spirits as we thought it would be fun to explore parts of the city we didn't know, so off we went, laughing and chatting.

Suddenly we were confronted by a policeman – what were we doing and what were our plans? Rather surprised at this meeting and the questioning we told him that we were just having a 'look-see'- at places we didn't know.

Our member of the law enforcement brigade very swiftly told us to follow him – we did, and he led us out of the notorious red light area to a more suitable region, accompanied with a few dire warnings and advice to stay away!

We were quite relieved to find we were safe after our little foray and soon found we were passing a fish and chip shop – the aroma was irresistible and we each had three pennyworth of chips – delicious! – we were celebrating!

Male Surgical Ward

Next day we looked at the notice board which was in the dining room, to see the ward of our first assignment. I was going to a massive fifty-odd bedded male surgical ward – rather a daunting thought. My first task was to sweep part of this large area – there must be no speck of dust or fluff remaining under the lockers or bed legs. Everywhere smelled strongly of disinfectant – a beautiful refreshing aroma, one I really appreciated and breathed in with pleasure. This would be especially liked in the future when I returned after a few days leave. I would feel back at home in the world I learned to love.

But I will continue with my first real duty – it demanded that I must walk to the opposite end of the ward avoiding many odd remarks from the patients and the occasional wolf whistle, and enter the sluice! Wow! Disinfectant was certainly the order of the day! A senior nurse came in and explained my first real taste of nursing training.

A very large double trolley stood in the centre of the room. It had to be filled with bed pans and urine bottles and I had to proceed to each bed with the trolley asking the occupant which receptacle – if any – they required. Some asked for toilet paper – No! we didn't supply such luxuries – but I did have tow. Now in case my reader doesn't know what tow is, I will endeavour to explain. It's a very coarse mixture of fibres and something like twigs – the whole thing resembling something gathered from beneath a prickly hedge. Without becoming too personal, I will just say it was hard on my hands as I supplied any poor misguided soul requiring it.

My mind boggled at the thought of the result of using this material on one's tender posterior area.

With my face getting redder by the minute, I

completed the 'giving out run' – now it was time to go back on the collection run – we'll quickly pass the details!

Eye Ward

My second placement was the eye ward – this was a very quiet ward with most patients lying flat with bandaged eyes.

Derby was in a mining area and we received several miners with eye injuries – it would sometimes be a shard of coal or iron that had pierced the eye and this demanded the most difficult of operations to remove the object.

Our eye surgeon was a truly lovely man and although all his operations required the utmost skill, he was always completely unruffled as he worked to save sight. In the eye theatre was a massive construction over the table – it was a huge light and a magnet. He would so deftly control the machine and he really worked what seemed to us real miracles as we watched.

One of the more usual correction eye operations was that of the strabismus – cross eyes. This was usually very successful and it was so lovely to watch the joy on the face of the patients as they looked into a mirror after about 10-14 days in bandages.

A side ward of four beds was kept for cataract patients. It was my duty to go into this ward as soon as I came on duty in the morning; I had to sweep and then swab the floor with disinfectant. Then I washed the four men who had received cataract operations. These men were all in their eighties and were all grand fellows. They never complained although they had to lie flat with a sandbag on either side of the head for ten days. Their only entertainment was a set of headphones. Of course they were unable to feed themselves and when I had prepared them for the day, all clean and spruce, another nurse would help me to feed them with breakfast. We always closed the door during the whole of the time I was in with them and we usually had a sing-along. It was a happy beginning to the day.

Night Duty and Babies

After the three months of happy and varied training on the Eye Ward, I was to go on night duty. My next ward was medical, consisting of one larger ward with maybe twenty patients and three or four side wards leading off the corridor – in one of which were five very sick small babies.

I was to give each one its nightly feed and hopefully after tucking them down, they would sleep. When five babies all decide it's time for choir practice, it's a sound which is better not heard. So I prayed that they would sleep – but first I must begin with the feeds.

I picked up my first little fellow – just a scrap of humanity so small and helpless – and sat down in the low nursing chair. He had been born with spina bifida. For the first half of his milk feed, he tucked in well and I felt pleased; after giving him the necessary minute or so to 'bring up his wind' I held him in my arms again in the feeding position – but somehow things were not right. I tried to encourage him to suck again – but without success. Suddenly the vein in his forehead began to bulge – I was scared, but before I could rise from the chair and seek assistance my little patient gasped and was gone. What a lovely little angel, I thought. I had experienced my first death and it would forever stay in my memory.

The effect of losing that wee bundle was shattering and I was utterly unable to stop trembling – with tears streaming down my face. Senior Night Sister had been called to the sad occurrence and immediately came in to me – she was a very large lady and she always took over the whole scene whatever was happening. She usually crisply gave her orders and everyone always humbly submitted to her voice. But this time she was different – kind and gracious to me, explaining that the death was caused by a cerebral haemorrhage – I could have done nothing to save him. Now I must behave in a professional manner – but at eighteen years of age this was rather difficult. Senior Night Nurse gave me a hot cup of tea and two aspirins and I was left alone with my thoughts for several minutes. I just longed to feel my mother's arms around me to comfort me – but she had died when I was eleven years old.

Night Sister walked in to me carrying a kidney dish complete with full syringe. "Now nurse," she said, "you are going to give Mrs So and So her midnight injection!" – somehow I managed to protest – I couldn't! I'd only ever given an injection to a model when in nursing school.

Sister looked me straight in the eye with those piercing eyes of hers and said, "Nurse, you are to obey orders". The glass syringe jingled in the enamel dish as we walked towards the patient.

I must pull myself together and stop trembling, otherwise I'd never be able to insert the needle. The patient was a sweet, kind, cuddly-type older woman, and she insisted that my injection was one of the best she had had since coming into hospital. I was very grateful to her, but suspected that Sister had had a prior chat with her.

There were five of our school on night duty so we always enjoyed getting together when we came off duty and going over our successes and failures – there were the inevitable tears and laughter, and how pleased we all were to be in the daylight.

The food in the hospital was appalling and somehow eating was our priority. As we came off duty, we would go into the ward kitchen and hack off a large chunk of bread from the loaf in the bread bin. Then we joined forces to see if any of us had generous patients! Sometimes it was a tomato, maybe two, or even an egg – now they were precious - or perhaps an apple or pear, or two cigarettes.

We took the loot to our kitchen in the Home and worked out the best way for ultimate use. It was fun and we enjoyed those 'get togethers', known as witches' brews. Rationing was severe and we were given only two ounces of butter each week for personal use, and two ounces didn't go far!

Days Off

Derby had a lovely little theatre and we would go along when the budget allowed. The price of a seat in the 'gods' was three shillings – fifteen pence in the twenty-first century.

We noticed that on one occasion the writer and actor Emlyn Williams was 'coming shortly' – we decided to try for 'off duty' and go along. During the first three days of the week 'The Corn is Green' was the production, and the second part of the week 'Night Must Fall'. In each Emlyn was playing the lead – it was all excellent and we were very pleased to get his autograph on our second visit. We all secretly wished he would be admitted to our hospital for something or other, but he was very hale and hearty and moved to his next city.

On one of our days off we decided to get up early and do two hours hard swatting – lectures and tests were an ever present evil and we had the end of a course of lectures and the exam just around the corner. But we had decided to go out and hopefully have a good day. At last we were ready and we collected our sandwiches from the main kitchen. We could have a picnic lunch if we gave sufficient advance notice – this was in lieu of our main lunch.

With merry hearts we stepped out to go by bus to the very beautiful part of Derbyshire known as The Dales. This was my first visit and I was thrilled. We wandered along by the River Dove – it was all so peaceful, only the odd fisherman. We made the mistake of brightly wishing them a 'good morning'. We learned that anglers do not appreciate this happy greeting. They like everything to be as silent as possible – ah well, we went on hiding our girlish giggles.

We clambered over hill and dale in the shadow of lovely Thorpe Cloud, and crossed the stepping stones – without anyone falling in – but soon felt the need for our picnic, so we chose an idyllic spot under a spreading tree and we lay back in the long grass. The sun was warm, the birds were singing, no one else around. The world was ours and what a wonderful world it was. We wished the day would never end.

But duty called! We were now young women anxious to show we meant to do the right thing. So we set off to catch the return bus. Strangely, a restaurant appeared unexpectedly on the brow of the hill overlooking some glorious countryside. There was a tariff on the wooden gateway, which was rather like an old five-barred farm gate. We read it, and one of the items was 'cup of tea and one teacake' – now that all sounded delicious and the price seemed fair. We produced our wealth. Had we enough for the yummy sounding refreshments and was there sufficient for our fare back to the city? Yes, it could be done, so we boldly walked in through the gate. Out of the posh restaurant emerged the obvious owner – black suit, white shirt, black tie and the immaculately folded napkin over his arm. He stood still – well you could say transfixed. His puckered forehead and worried eyes scanned us from head to toe. Our apparel did nothing to cheer him, we were thoroughly scruffy after our lovely day of roaming the hills and dales – but at least our hands and faces were clean; we had washed those in the stream. He asked us what we were thinking of ordering – no, it wasn't the five-course meal which sounded scrumptious, didn't rationing exist around here? Feeling very humble in the great man's presence, we quietly breathed "a cup of tea and one teacake please for each of us". Now this had to be mulled over for what seemed an eternity. Then a very begrudging "all right" passed from those tight lips –

"but don't come into the dining room – your order will be placed on the wooden tables outside". We were highly amused at all this and sat down on the hard wooden seats and hoped the cushions and pretty table cloth would maybe follow – hopes were unfulfilled – but the refreshment was lovely and we all tucked in.

The great chief must have been observing us from his inner sanctuary as he immediately appeared to collect our money as soon as the last crumb was consumed. He then thankfully prepared to show us to the gate – but not so swift. Joyce gracefully extended her hand and stopped him in his tracks. "We all happen to be nurses at the Royal," she said, "and should you ever find the need to come to our hospital for help we'll remember to ask you where you would like your bed to be placed".

We felt that we had won the deciding round and headed along the lane with light hearts and faces wreathed in smiles. It had been a day long to be remembered.

Just outside Derby was a large American Air Force base. From the airfield the huge Flying Fortress bombers flew to bomb targets in Europe.

We would watch as they flew out in tight formation on their mission. The sight of these huge aircraft flying low over our city as they gradually gained height with their massive loads brought mixed feelings – they were doing a splendid job – trying eventually to cause peace to come. We always wondered how many young men would fly back over our hospital – and how the formations would look then – it was a sobering thought.

Women's Medical Ward

I was now working on a women's medical ward, and I have already commented earlier on the standard of food throughout the establishment. One day each week the main course at lunch was a concoction known with the all-embracing title of 'mash' – this was corned beef and mashed potatoes well mixed with gravy. Now at this time in the 1940s there was a great desire to whip out children's tonsils for all sorts of complaints. We had one day each week which was allotted to tonsil removals. Strangely enough the mash day always followed tonsil day – now I'm not suggesting any connection but I think you would agree with the nickname given to the tasteless offering placed on each plate in the form of a 'dollop' – not even a cabbage leaf to cheer the look of this delicacy – it was named 'tonsil mash'.

The women patients on our ward were a merry crew – the type it's a real joy to nurse. What we on the staff didn't know was that three of them had held a 'council of war' with their husbands at visiting time and it was placed in the hands of these three trusty men to inform the Board of Governors about the offending 'mash'.

Well, the day came for the unwelcome offering on a plate again.

We had finished serving and were enduring the usual remarks along with suggestions for what to do with it! Some plates were just as we had delivered them, others showed that the women were made of stern stuff and had sampled it.

So the rubbish bin in the ward kitchen was rapidly becoming full. Now, it was at this point that the phone rang and after taking the call, Sister came into the kitchen and said with her eyes sparkling, "We are to have a visit immediately from three members of the Board. They wish to have a helping of mash!" This sounded like a tricky situation - oh well, only one thing to do – we hastily prepared three trays with plates and cutlery. At this point we should take precautions and we closed the kitchen door; sightseers were not welcome! Then we proceeded to take a dollop out of the rubbish bin and place this delicately on each plate, doing our best to make the tasty morsel look attractive. I must now say that we had never heard of Edwina Currie and salmonella, which was just as well.

Then Sister collected them and delivered them to the prestigious visitors.

Strangely enough we never did get any 'feedback' but mash was then always missing from the menu.

Life continued slowly, we were changed from one ward to another to widen our experience and training.

Odd Jobs

Personally I was longing for the day when I'd pass my first national examination and so move up a step or so, as I found the endless rounds of distribution and recovery of bed pans rather an unpleasant pastime, which of course was followed by the everlasting scrubbing and clearing out of the aforementioned necessary articles, not really to my taste of entertainment.

Then there was the everlasting lower back and buttocks rubbing of every patient confined to bed, to be done with soapy hands – then very careful drying and finally a tiny spot of meths – this was all to prevent bed sores – it was a 4-hourly chore and woe betide the nurse allowing a patient to have a bed sore – nurses had to attend a kind of court martial in Sister's presence if this happened – so it was beneficial to all concerned to rub well and so increase the blood supply and reduce the pressure.

On night duty we had a much more pleasant task – flowers – and there were a lot, as in those days flowers were considered a benefit to patients. All the vases had to be washed and flowers sorted and re-arranged – this all happened in the flower room, the scent of which was a great improvement to some places.

Arranging the flowers was fun – some nurses were very gifted with powers of decoration and would have made good florists if their nursing career failed.

But we must not take too long with the flowers – other duties awaited us and there was often the call from a wide awake patient needing help. Sewing was the next work, and we had abdominal bandages to make – these consisted of a central large piece of material to which we had to sew tails – that meant long pieces of bandage being sewn across the central part leaving long tails either side which when it had become a finished article could be used for abdominal wounds and the tails were tied at the side and back. Really they looked rather like an octopus and I doubt if they were very comfortable.

Then there were the poultices to make – now to do this a piece of linen was taken, about twelve inches square, with a thick layer of kaolin spread over, topped off with muslin, then the sides of linen were folded in.

These poultices were packed carefully and put away until needed. They were then warmed up in the kitchen oven and the intention was to bring comfort when applied to painful areas. Care had to be taken not to burn the patient.

Then of course there was the sluice to be thoroughly cleaned – walls and all – so that everything was in order for the dawning of a new day.

Patient Care

But night duty was a rewarding time. There were normally two nurses on each ward at night and every little while one of us would walk silently round the beds to observe every patient. We would notice some of them awake and restless; immediately we went alongside the bed to enquire as to what was wrong. Sometimes it was physical pain which could be relieved with a more comfortable position and a warm drink and tablet to relieve the pain. But sometimes it was different – they were worried and deeply concerned – mothers had left their children at home or with grandparents or friends, all of whom were trying to fill in for the missing mum, but children often get so upset and play up badly for attention as they long for their beloved parent again.

Then fathers who were facing long stays in hospital – probably for the first time in their lives – were worried over financial affairs – how will the family manage or would they lose their job? When it was money difficulties we could always arrange a visit from the Almoner next day.

As we listened intently and spoke in whispers, remembering that other patients were asleep, we realised that although we were personally unable to put the situation right, often just listening seemed to help the troubled soul and after a while the patient would relax a little; we felt pleased and would wipe the tears, rearrange the pillow, give a hug, then a warm drink, and pray that the patient would be able to sleep. Usually it was so rewarding to notice that after a while restful sleep had come and with it some degree of healing of mind and body.

Now this was what nursing was all about!

One day I was delayed in leaving the ward and arrived rather late in the dining room for lunch. Now I must explain how seating was arranged in the aforementioned room – first the very junior pros sat together on two large tables, then the slightly higher nursing ranks and finally the tables at which sat junior then finally senior staff nurses and never the twain must meet between lowly pros and senior staff until this day when I was arriving late.

In panic I looked around for a vacant chair – and then was directed to a place at the senior staff's table. Well, this was awful – they all gave me a threatening look and I sat down with trepidation and gave a longing glance towards the juniors' tables.

Somehow my appetite had gone but I coped with the first course and then the dessert was served – it was a tart – well actually a square piece of pastry topped with blackcurrants in a sauce – quite good – but the base was very difficult to cut and I was trying valiantly with my fork when suddenly the whole sweet took off and landed on the plate of the staff nurse sitting opposite. Oh the humiliation! She swiftly lifted her plate demanding (it seemed to me in an unnecessarily loud voice – so that the whole assembly was made aware) that this plate be removed and a fresh one brought to her. No one brought me another helping and I felt this was a blessing.

At last the signal came that we might leave and I thankfully joined my pals to recuperate.

Exams

Time was moving on and the National Nursing Examination was upon us. We lived through the written tests – but the practical was different. This was held in another hospital across town – now that was a bad start! No hospital was as good as the Royal. We were lost in the many corridors and no-one seemed to help – it wouldn't have happened at the Royal! Finally we were directed to a large hall.

Our names were called and we went in two at a time…

As we entered we noticed two Matrons standing at the far end of the hall, and quite a distance it was too – or so it seemed. We were instructed as to which Matron was ours, and off we went. 'My' Matron watched my every movement as I walked towards her. Did I give the appearance of confidence and would patients feel they were in safe hands? Well, all I knew just then was that my legs were full of jelly and my heart beat was well above an acceptable rate. I was eventually standing before this navy clad person who greeted me with an icy, "Good morning, Nurse". Life began in earnest with a barrage of questions which I thought lasted for hours, but by glancing at the large wall clock showed a mere ten minutes – had the clock stopped?

Next I was to collect a metal tray and place on it bowls and various instruments of torture such as an enema syringe and other necessary implements. I then had to carry them back to a large table and set them out for dressings and operations as instructed.

Unfortunately, just as I was carrying these items to the table, there was a terrific crash just behind me. I was later to learn that my friend had dropped her full tray onto the quarry tiled floor. The quiet of the hall was shattered but I knew I must remain undisturbed and not look round, all this was not conducive to effortless decorum.

Somehow the part for trays was over – now it was on to showing our bandaging skills. Now bandaging was never one of my brighter spots!

My model was a soldier recruited from one of the wards – which was a reasonably easy task!

Matron informed me I was to bandage the head as if he was suffering from post operative double mastoid. That was a rather unkind choice of bandage I felt, why not a cut thumb or something similar?

I had a limited time in which to complete this new fashion accessory. My 'model' was highly amused – he was having fun and being paid for it, even if it was a mere pittance – and was full of non-stop useful hints to make the perfect bandage. After a few minutes Matron came to examine the said object, "yes it looked good,", it covered the whole head well with special emphasis on the ears! But was it comfortable and did it feel secure and would it offer protection for the post operative ears? Matron directed the questions to my model. "Absolutely perfect, feels so comfortable," came the reply – so with a nod of approval Matron said I could now remove my work of art – "and rewind the bandage as you go". I breathed again. As soon as my examiner was on her way back to her position, my model just lifted the whole concoction from his head and handed it to me! I was furious – there was no need for him to announce to the world how badly fitting was my work. I quickly pushed it back on to his curly locks, they may look good but were little value as an anchor, he was tickled pink – I was breathing out death threats through clenched teeth. Although he was really quite a good looking fellow, it was easy to go off people!

At long last the hour was completed and we went back to normal duties to await our results.

Chapter Two

Illness Strikes

It was about this time that I began to feel rather unwell, all my joints were very swollen and I was in much pain – I had a form of rheumatism and I was confined to bed for some time.

Treatment continued and gradually I began to feel better and the pain was less. I wondered when I would return to duty. One morning Home Sister came in on her usual round, but this time was accompanied by the medical officer for nurses. I was duly examined once more and after some minutes of hushed talk between my visitors they returned to my bedside looking very sombre. "Yes, Nurse, you are improving but now you must face the fact that you will never be fit enough to nurse again". Then Sister piped up with the awful news, "You must vacate your room as soon as possible – preferably tomorrow!" They both wished me good luck and closed the door – I was alone.

Now, my sister and I both began our nursing careers at the same time, but not at the same hospital. She had settled in another Midlands town and we kept in very close contact with each other. It had been an awful wrench to part and go our separate ways, but she was four years older than me and I always felt that she was endowed with more brain power than her younger sister, as a result I was always in her shadow, and was certain that if we had gone to the same establishment I would probably have been a source of embarrassment to her – hence our choice of separate hospitals.

But today I needed her badly – I was soon in touch and she came to me next day. Knowing that the situation at home was rather difficult – my father and his new wife had a small child, and therefore a rather unwell lass would not be very welcome, I decided to ring a very old and dear friend to ask for help. She immediately came to my aid and so it was that the next day I packed my case and with a heavy heart began to make the journey of departure, but first I must call at the office to collect certain papers. Sister handed them over, then demanded the return of my 'Student Nurse' badge and returned to me the one shilling and three pence.

This really hurt to hand over my badge. I walked back through the gateway and down the grimy street which led to the station. I had no real home to which I could go – just that of a friend – no job or hope of one, and a few health problems yet to be resolved. I felt devastated but pulling my shoulders back made up my mind to somehow win through.

With sad farewells to chums ringing in my ears, I at last arrived at my friend's home. There I received a big hug and an assurance that "we'll soon get you well". Her husband was serving in the Forces and she had two lovely little boys whom I dearly loved, and I was in that happy home for the next seven months or so.

There was just one thing which I found very annoying there. A siren had been placed strategically on a building nearby. Now I knew that sirens were very necessary to warn of enemy aircraft approaching – but the actual sound was deafening. Somehow of course the 'all clear' never seemed quite so bad, maybe it was because of the message it announced.

I must explain that shortage of money played quite a part in my life. I had one pair of black duty shoes and one pair of quiet soled sandals for night duty, but apart from that only one pair of mufti shoes and they were very well worn and beyond repair so I had to push cardboard into the shoe as the sole – this made for little comfort when walking on rough surfaces and also wet feet if it rained, and I was constantly on the lookout for cardboard. One day my friend casually said that she was walking into the village to do some shopping – would I care to join her? Yes, that sounded good. The village was quite upmarket and had a few very attractive shops with excellent quality wares. As we walked along, my friend said she mainly wished to purchase some shoes as she was going to a special occasion. The little shop was lovely – thick carpet covered the whole area and the assistants were charming. I sat and watched the choice of shoes – a lovely beige – they were sweet and would look fine on the outing, then I heard the words casually spoken "There's a nice pair over there which would suit you!" My heart leapt – they were a super pair of brown leather – well of course the outcome was that I walked out of the shop wearing brand new shoes and carrying a paper bag with worn out footwear which was quickly popped into the nearest litter bin. My feet seemed airborne, and my heart was bursting with thanks which were quickly passed over. Now I knew the real mission of our shopping foray.

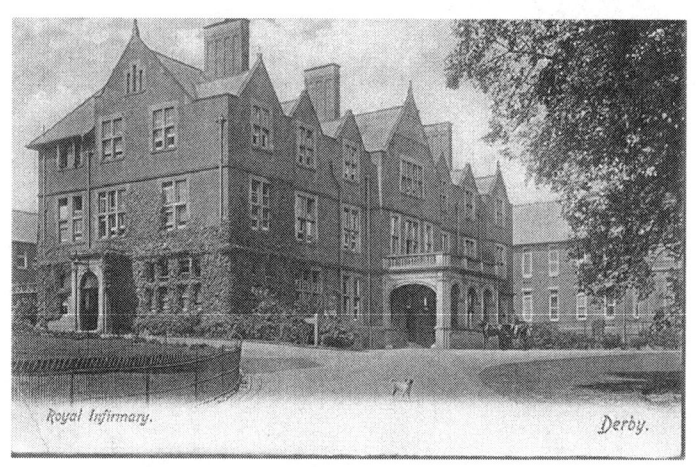

Derby Royal Infirmary Nurses School

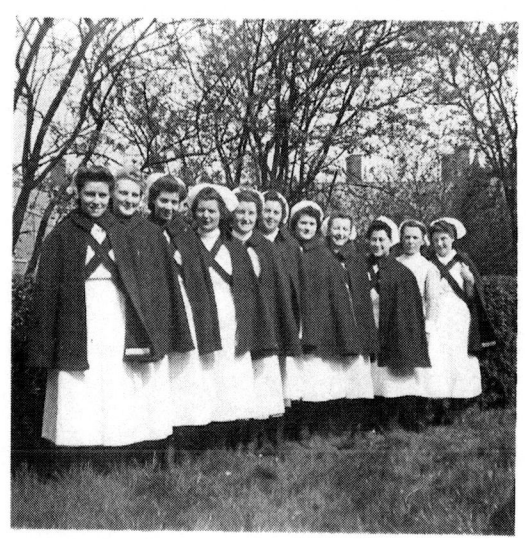

Derby Royal Infirmary Student Nurses

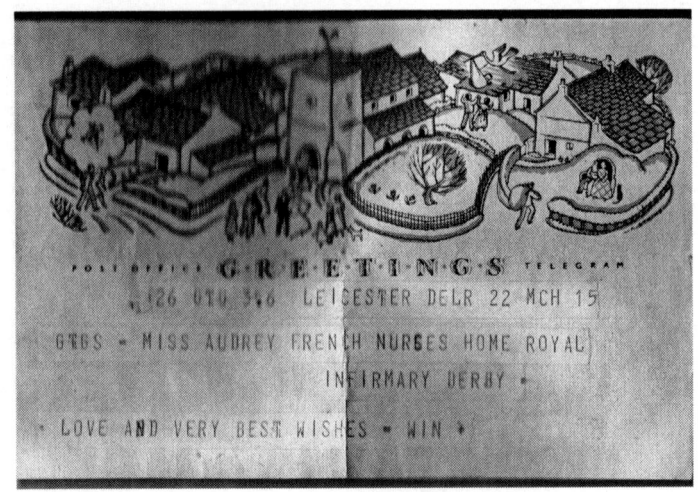

*Telegram from my sister Win
as I started training in Derby*

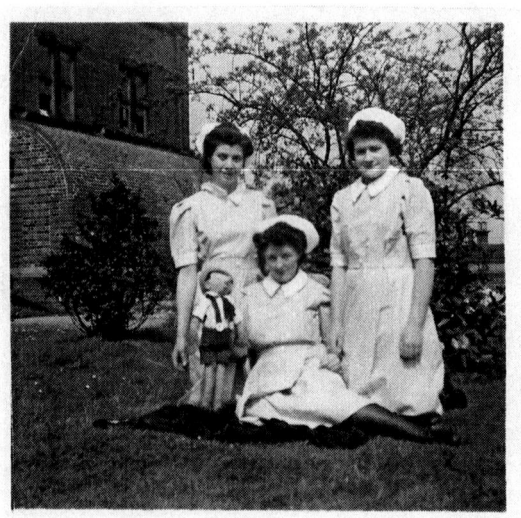

Forney, Kerby and Audrey

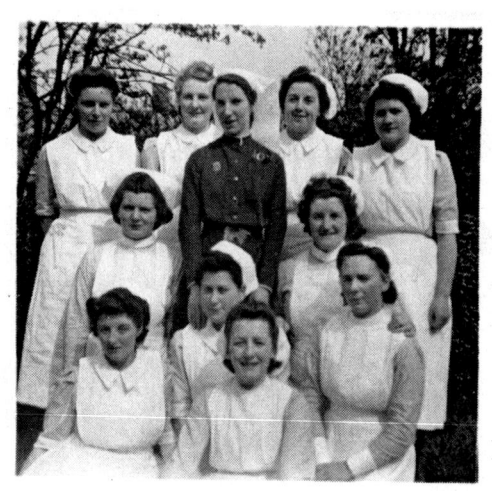

Derby Nurses with Sister Barton

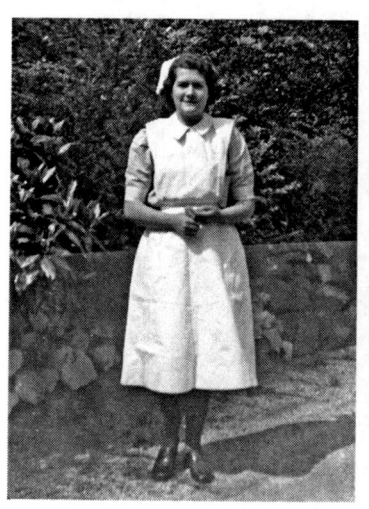
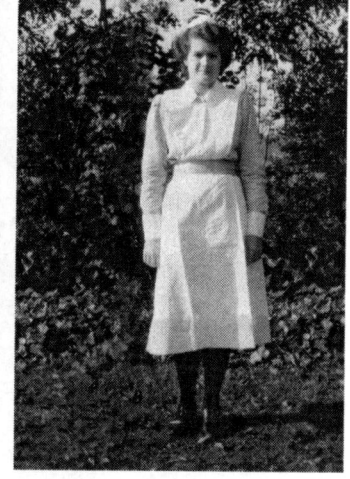

Nurse French

Derby Royal
(short sleeves —
in training)

West Herts
(long sleeves —
training completed)

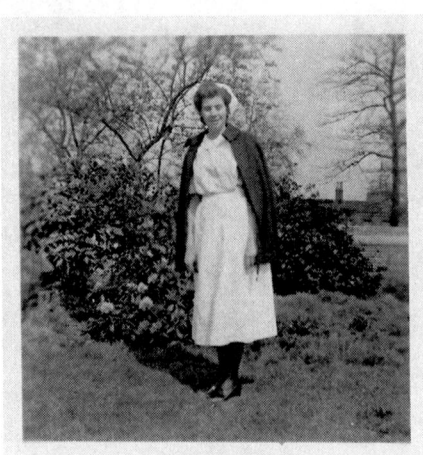

Kerby

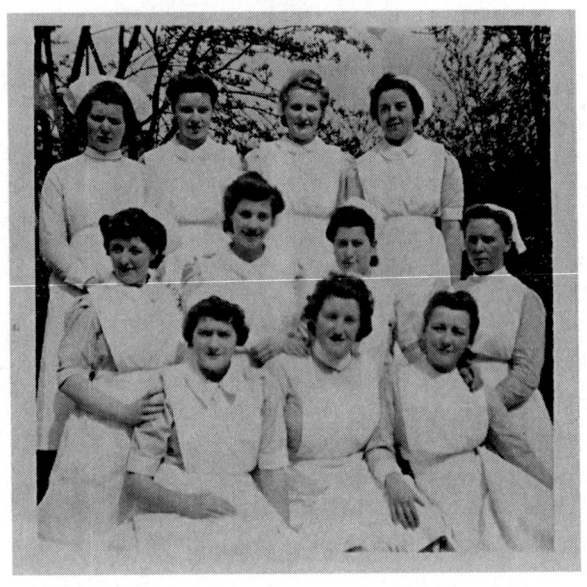

*Nurses Shipton, Saunders, Donkin, Shires,
Forney, Kerby, Amalan, Wood,
French, Stewart, Faulconbridge*

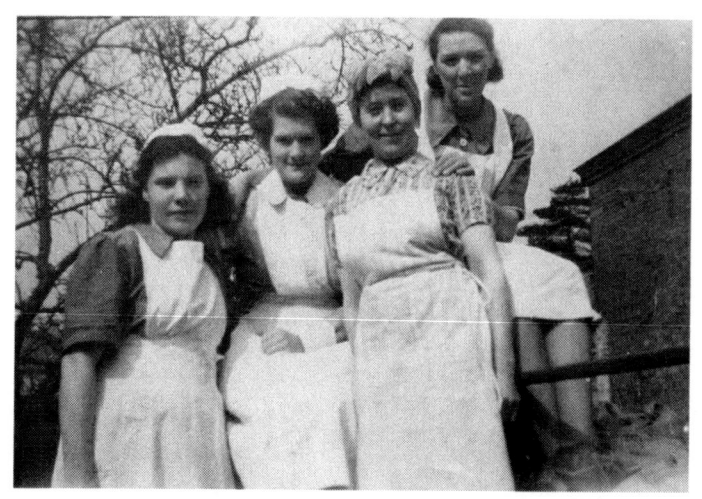

Keeping on good terms with the kitchen staff

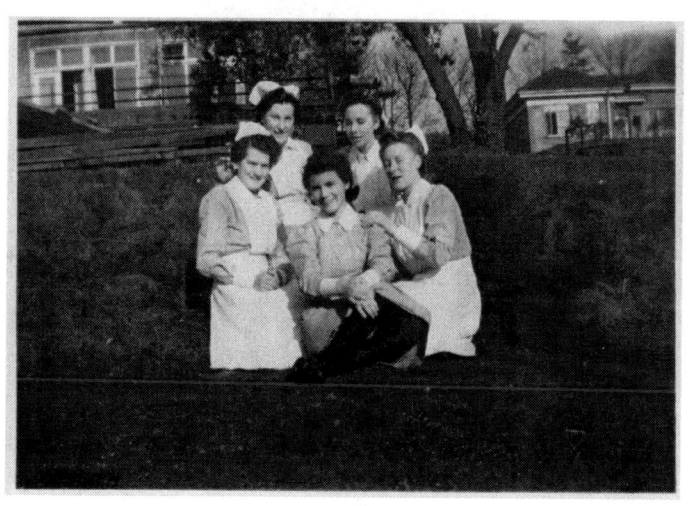

Friends

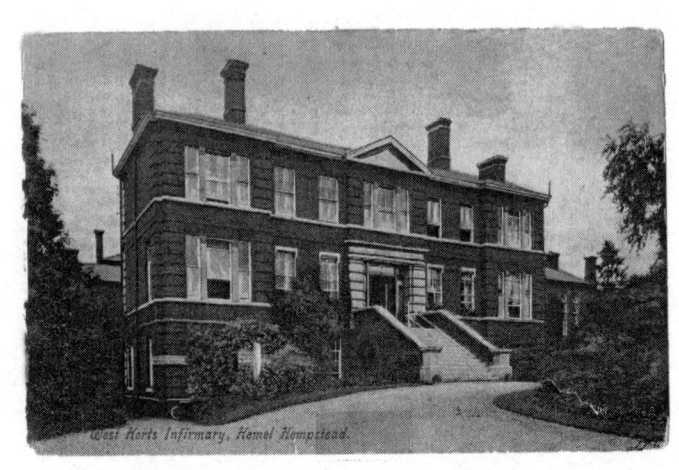

West Herts Hospital

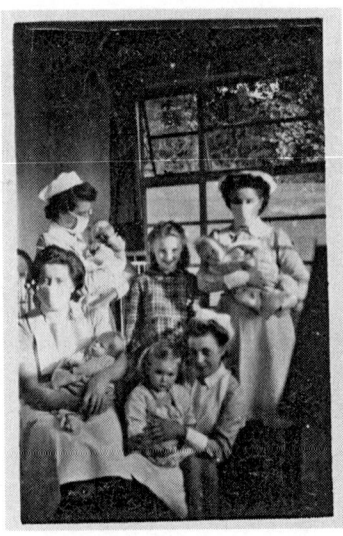

Children's Ward at West Herts Hospital

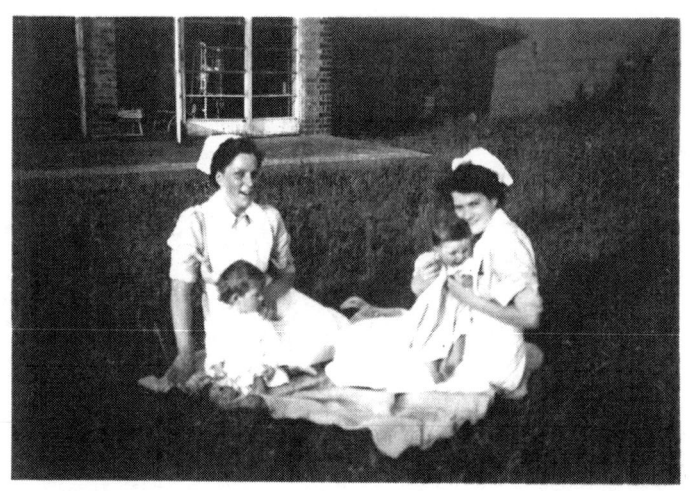

Beau and Audrey

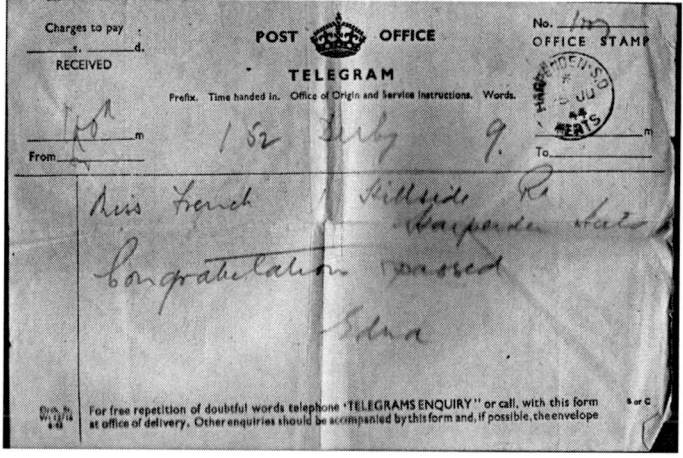

Telegram from Edna on my success at passing preliminary training.

Chapter Three

Starting Again
West Herts Hospital Hemel Hempstead

So time went by very pleasantly and my health was improving. After about four months I decided I must try to return to nursing. I wrote all around the country, but it was no good, as soon as my medical report was read I was rejected. Finally I tried a small rural hospital in a quiet town and I was thrilled when I read that I was being considered and would I attend for an interview and medical examination. Both the Home Sister and a Medical Officer were helpful and reassuring; yes they would accept me on three conditions, a three-monthly blood test, a six-monthly x-ray, they were fine. The third was the worst as I also had to agree to sleep between flannelette sheets. Now flannelette sheets at that time were made of a thick unbleached material which contained prickly bits of fibre entwined with the whole and made for rather an uncomfortable surface. Still that was nothing – I joyfully accepted – I was back.

So the day came and I was off to my new abode, with another hug from my friend and lots of good wishes.

Training Again

The new hospital was much smaller than my previous one, but straightway there was a friendly feeling pervading. Soon I realised that other girls had come along with various health reasons for leaving their previous hospitals – this was very encouraging.

So the morning arrived for the first day of duty here – I carefully arranged my rich auburn hair under the cap after donning my crisp new uniform – looked into the mirror and gave myself full marks and went along to breakfast, where of course I met other staff, and noted that I was being sent to the maternity ward.

Before going to the wards, all nurses went to the little chapel for morning prayers led by a Senior Sister.

Maternity Ward

The maternity ward was a new and happy experience for me and I was to be present at the next birth, a beautiful baby girl. The thrill of observing this wonderful happening was a very emotional moment as I realised what a marvellous work of creation is shown in a new addition to the human race – I'll thoroughly enjoy my time on this ward – yet there was to be one of the most terrifying moments to come.

Walking past the nursery one morning I heard a strange and alarming sound – a baby was choking. I rushed in, there were about twelve to fifteen babies at any time in there – one little lad was quite the leader in the weight stakes – a very chubby eleven pounds or so – now he was purple and choking. I grabbed him by the ankles and ran up the corridor carrying him upside down to the room where I knew Sister was. She was a midwife of many years experience. Swiftly placing a tiny tube into his mouth and down his throat, she withdrew the offending fluid. The little boy's colour slowly turned from purple to pink – he was breathing properly again – what a wonderful relief. Sister tipped him right way up and after several minutes of checking him she placed him in my arms with, "Well done Nurse, you have saved a little life".

Little did I know that a similar experience would occur over thirty years later on – the difference? It was now my precious grandson who was choking in my arms – but thankfully again it ended in a happy result. Caring for babies is great fun but also has its scary moments.

The Dining Hall was a friendly gathering place with lots of chatter and laughter. But there was just one thorn – there was a large top table at which dined the Sisters. One of the hospital rules was that whenever a Sister entered the Hall, nurses must stand, showing respect. Well, that was all right if the meal had not commenced, but if we had just filled a spoon with soup or with spaghetti or something similar and had arranged the fork suitably, we had to stand, trying to pop the aforementioned into the beginning of our digestive system, and push our chairs back at the same time, the chair loudly scraping the wooden floor. Then, of course, after the Sister had acknowledged our efforts with a "thank you nurses" the chairs were replaced with all the noise again and we recommenced our meal. No-one bothered to object – it was all part of life's rich tapestry.

Christmas on the Wards

Christmas was approaching and with it, all the joy of anticipation. Now hospital Sisters were all the same – they had a knack of saving scraps of fat and sugar from the meagre ward rations throughout the year to use in the sweet making production. No 'Best Before' in those days! For the general public sweets were strictly rationed, but our hospital wizards produced toffee apples, fudge, peppermint creams and chocolate drops, and the threats to anyone who dared to try to 'nick' a sample were very real.

Wards were decorated and the whole hospital became charged with a feeling of excitement and no one asked for time off over Christmas; we couldn't miss the happy season.

On Christmas Eve after we came off duty, one of the highlights of the festivities took place. All the nursing staff had navy cloaks lined with an eye-catching scarlet material, and every available nurse, with cloaks turned to the 'red', carried lighted lanterns and went from ward to ward, lights dimmed everywhere. The Assistant Matron was the musical mystic and played the piano – every ward had a piano – no T.V. in those days, and we all sang our hearts out with the carols. By each bed which contained a really sick patient would be a nurse just watching carefully, but patients who felt well enough joined in the singing and the throb of carols continued along corridors and wards Christmas had arrived, and it was just lovely.

Now on Christmas morning, the task of the junior nurse – that was me – was to prepare the coffee and mince pies. Our Ward Sister was very good at being organised and she had prepared the coffee beforehand to make sure it was just perfect. She had placed the prepared liquid in a large white enamel jug and at the appointed time the jug was to be placed in a saucepan of boiling water and brought up to the desired heat. Everything was going well; the coffee jug was put to warm up at exactly the right time and my thoughts turned to heating the oven ready to warm the mince pies, but there was a queer aroma around. Still I had other things to do and I left the kitchen to carry on by itself. Then, as the smell increased and drifted down to the main ward and all the side rooms, staff began to laugh and squiggle their noses - the place was smelling like a brewery!

I went back to check the kitchen and then the truth was made known – in the cupboard was another white enamel jug, it should have been containing the ale for lunchtime consumption, I'd chosen the wrong jug and was boiling the ale instead of the coffee. You can imagine the teasing I received when I went to the evening supper meal in the nurses' dining room. I found that the hospital grapevine was working well and I was greeted with laughter.

Christmas Day lunch was a very happy occasion – decorations everywhere, crackers (usually hand-made), and all the usual trimmings we could muster to go with the turkey. The roasted bird was brought in to the main part of each ward with great pomp and ceremony by one of the surgeons or physicians, sometimes dressed as a chef, who had come in especially to carve. Everything possible was done to give the patients a happy and memorable Christmas Day.

Sometimes of course there were emergency admissions, needing operations, and we always felt this was rather thoughtless.

But Christmas doesn't last long and we had to continue normal nursing activities.

Men's Medical on Nights

As the war was still on, accommodation became a problem for patients and staff alike. We needed two more wards and so Nissan huts had been erected. Nissan huts were made of wood and tin, painted black – with creosote I imagine – the smell was pretty potent. The roofs were made of corrugated iron and birds seemed to love running up and down them wearing wooden clogs – or so it sounded. A pokey little shed affair was added at one end, which went under the title of a kitchen, then a similar building called the sluice was also added. Our modern Health and Safety Officers would have had great fun sorting that out! Beds were closely arranged with only just room for a locker in between.

I was now becoming more of a senior nurse as I was gradually passing exams and tests.

I had met some lovely girls here and had formed friendships with one or two special friends which would last for years – there is Beau a great lass with whom I keep in constant touch, even after sixty years.

Night duty came around again and I was senior on the men's medical ward which was housed in one of the huts. We had some very sick patients. Three or four had breathing troubles due to heart weakness and they all had oxygen masks affixed to their faces, with huge canisters of oxygen standing beside them. It had taken a long while to get the ward quiet for the night and I was anxious about several of the men. At last the lights were dimmed and there was some degree of peace and a few contented snores!

Suddenly the silence was shattered – the nurse from the adjoining hut had popped in to borrow something, but in the dim light she didn't notice the fire extinguisher and had given it a hefty kick. Of course this had activated the extinguisher and the foam went everywhere accompanied with all the usual noise of the happening, the hissing seemed endless. Patients were leaping up in their beds in horror – oxygen masks were torn off – those on drips had pulled the tubes out, asthma patients started attacks – it was mayhem. We put all the lights on as we tried to explain it was all fine – just a fire extinguisher doing its normal – no, it wasn't the end of the world. It took quite a time to settle our patients back – masks etc in situ again. Junior had the good idea of putting on the kettle – it's wonderful what a cuppa can do.

Now we found we had the simple matter of cleaning up the floor – just how far can foam travel? Eventually we began to see the funny side of the occurrence and that always helps and gradually everyone settled once more, and it seemed that dawn broke early that morning.

Nights were always rather hectic on this ward and on one occasion we were very sad. Two men had died in the small hours of the night, my poor junior was very upset at having to 'lay out the patient', it was a great ordeal for her. This is thankfully not carried out in hospital now and is confined to the funeral parlour.

Time was running out – we'd been very busy and there was much more to do before the day staff would arrive. I suggested that if she would go round and clean the dentures, I would give out the medicines and we'd join up to wash our patients – it was going well. I'd almost finished medicines when she came to me and said "I'm in trouble" – and she was! She was carrying a bowl full of water and all the dentures for the whole ward!!! Now if you have every tried fitting a jigsaw together, I think you'll understand. We were glad when the day staff came on duty and our night was over.

Friends

During this time I was very fond of what seemed to me, the most wonderful young man – I'd known him for a long while and he filled my thoughts at every possible waking hour. It was just lovely to be in his presence and I watched the post daily looking for his handwriting which would lift me all day. Then the morning came when I received a note which was to tell me that he wished to end our friendship. For some long time, I felt my heart would break, but hearts do heal eventually even if there is always that tiny part which never really does recover completely.

I stuffed the letter into my pocket and walked into the ward – I was on duty!

My friend, Beau, had been unwell for some weeks, although carried on with her duties. It was decided that her tonsils must be removed. Arrangements were made for her to be cared for in a small room containing the sterile water units as there was no private ward available. The day came for the tonsillectomy – things did not go well and Beau haemorrhaged badly and had to return to theatre. She was very poorly for some days. I spent all my off duty time sitting with her and when on duty it was amazing how many times we needed sterile water – I would pop off to Beau's little room and then hide it in my apron. On another visit I would return it to the shelves. There is a limit to the amount of water needed on just one ward.

At last Beau was fit enough to return home to recuperate and I missed her so much and looked forward to her coming back to hospital to nurse again.

Senior nurses were now being housed in the Nissan huts erected to relieve the pressure for nurses' rooms in the main Home. We could all be trusted (how mistaken can hierarchy be?) to be in by 10.30 pm. Night Sister came around at that time and ceremoniously locked the outer door of the sitting room.

The huts were arranged as a threesome – two were sleeping quarters and the other hut joined them and formed the bathroom, kitchen and sitting room and it was in the latter that we kept a tiny book with the names of anyone planning to come in late without obtaining a late pass, of course. So, as soon as Sister disappeared we remedied the situation by unlocking the door. Sometimes there was quite a little list of erring nurses and occasionally the door was never locked again – they were happy days. However, there was one girl who was a pest, thoroughly dictatorial and causing so much annoyance that action was needed. So we ran a bath of cold water, waited until all was quiet in the offender's room, then we pounced and picked her up in her lovely pink organza nightie – we were all jealous! The nightie had been sent to her by an uncle in the U.S.A. some years earlier; we'd heard every chapter and verse about it! We dumped her in the bath and disappeared to our beds. Somehow she got the message and turned out to be a really nice person – obviously cold baths have therapeutic properties.

Life and Death

Following the normal duty time on one ward we were moved to another and this time for me it was to the women's medical ward in the other Nissan hut.

It was a busy ward and we were without antibiotics and the many drugs which would be used in coming years, so patients were often in for long stays and we came to know them and their visitors very well.

We had an emergency admission – a lass of eighteen years old. She had a tooth abscess which had burst and sent poison throughout her body; general septicaemia. She was desperately ill and begged to see her fiancé, a soldier serving somewhere in Europe. It was decided to try to contact him – phone calls were dashed around and he was flown in from the continent, but she was so ill – everything possible was done to hold on to her until he came, but bless her, she died a few minutes before he walked in to be by her side – there were no dry eyes anywhere that day.

Everything possible was cleaned and disinfected from top to bottom when a patient died or was discharged.

On this ward we had wooden lockers and they were always well scrubbed at such an opportunity.

We had one nurse who was very zealous and decided to take two lockers out through the door and give them a good cleaning outside. Fair enough – it was a lovely day and we tried to use the garden space whenever we could and mobile patients were glad to sit out there.

We thought the cleaning was going well and took no notice until we heard shouting – Nurse Postlewaite had decided to sterilise by means of methylated spirit and a lighted match! Well, at least, she had a successfully sterile locker – even if wood ash is not much use beside a bed!

Ups and Downs

Days went swiftly by and we were always very busy. One lovely lady in her 80s had come in following a stroke which left her partly paralysed, the physiotherapist was often encouraging movement, and we never heard any complaints, and we loved helping her to move her hands a little. She was especially fond of chocolate and would quite often ask for two squares of the goodie. Now good chocolate was difficult to obtain – but her two lovely daughters somehow kept up a well stocked little box of chocolate for their mother. When she asked in her sweet way for "two squares, please, Nurse" we would place them just a centimetre or so past her fingers and she would struggle until she could reach them and with eyes shining would tell us she'd done it! Dear Edna – the day came for her to go to live with her daughters, as she went she turned and said, "You know, patients have to get better here – it's just such a happy place". Yes, it was largely true – but not quite always.

Our young registrar was a very good looking lively young man and the patients all enjoyed a visit from him.

One day he asked to see a certain visitor because he was anxious to speak about a sick relative. The arrangement was made for the meeting and they stood outside the ward chatting. The visitor was a young attractive woman and she and the doctor were in deep discussion when suddenly we noticed pale blue French silk panties descending which fell to the floor – our lass just bent down, picked up the pretty underwear and popped it into her pocket, without either of them breaking off the conversation. We felt it was something very neatly carried out – we were going to store that for future reference if ever needed!

Another sweet patient was suffering from advanced cancer and we knew she was unlikely to recover and there was none of the advanced treatment of the 21st century available. She felt that a sprig of rosemary tucked into her bandage would help the healing process. Ward Sister was a very firm individual and insisted the rosemary be removed, causing much distress, which we felt was unnecessary – we all knew the prognosis was very poor, so when Sister went off duty we would place the rosemary back in the required position and it helped those last few weeks so much.

A sergeant from the Army was admitted with a perforated appendix. He was very sick, but still carried on shouting out orders as if on the parade ground.

After the operation he begged for a drink of water, he was given the usual glass with instructions to only sip the water. He was a bad-tempered man in his 40s, and promptly drank all the water in one swallow, we warned him about being silly and that he would probably be sick, and this was dangerous for his newly sewn wounds. He carried on demanding water and eventually was given a full jug, he just picked it up and gulped all the contents. Of course, he was violently sick and fell back on his pillows exhausted. Concern was felt about his stitches – had they burst? No, all was fine, and by the evening time he was hale and hearty and walking around – something unheard of in those days. We all felt that maybe having copious drinks after an operation was probably a pretty good idea. He discharged himself the next day, much to the relief of all the staff.

The Theatre

I knew that it was time for me to move on, and I had an awful dread that it might be general operating theatre, and one morning going into the dining room, I glanced at the notice board – yes, there it was – my next assignment commencing that day was theatre! Well that was the end of any breakfast for me, I could not tolerate the thought of three months in theatre; there must be a way out. Surely the 'powers that be' had made a complete mistake. Walking along the long corridor, I was practising my speech! No way was theatre for me etc etc – I had many reasons. Sisters always came on duty an hour later than other staff. I waited impatiently until at last Sister appeared – a dynamic little body with a ready smile and big blue eyes. She had served for a while, or so the gossip said, with the Desert Rats in Africa, but had been sent back to England for health reasons; well right now, as she called me into the office, she appeared extremely fit.

She welcomed me to theatre and said she had read my reports from other wards and knew I'd be very happy and capable as a theatre nurse – well, we all make mistakes! Before I could begin my speech she continued – "I see from your face that you do not agree with me – come back to my office a week today and we'll have another chat." With that she showed me the door. Chat? I had had no chance to say a word. I was soon being told by a senior how to prepare the theatre for the operation due to take place shortly.

Wow! There was no escape hatch. As the week went by I found myself settling down and actually enjoying the bustle of it all – I say 'bustle' but that doesn't mean panic, it was all so efficiently maintained. Every tile in the theatre was cleaned and disinfected at the beginning of the day and again between each op; the whole place was scrupulously clean and smelled lovely – so clinical. The instruments were kept in glass cases in the theatre walls. I had to learn the names and uses of each instrument. During an operation, swabs of linen gauze-like material were used for mopping up – so operations were clean and non-gory.

Swabs were placed in tens and as each pack was opened a mark was made on a large board. This board contained hooks which were all numbered – 1 to 10.

As each swab was used and then discarded, we would arrange it on a hook and so continue until all ten hooks were full. Then another mark would be made indicating all swabs had been retrieved from the incision – it's rather important not to leave a 'foreign body' in the patient – unthinkable.

There was a great feeling of camaraderie amongst theatre staff. I noticed that some surgeons were quite jovial throughout whilst others were quiet and I was beginning to get the drift. There was much eye contact over the masks. Life was coming good.

The latest recruit to theatre was always considered the junior – gradually ascending the scale as we gained experience.

The time appointed came at the end of the first week for my visit to Sister's office. This was a different 'me' walking through the door. She greeted me with an amused smile. "I was right, wasn't I nurse?" she said. How right she was – we chatted for a minute or so and then she wished me a happy three months of theatre training. How well she judged me – I was to love those days.

Important Visitors

It was the duty of the junior nurse to tie the gowns of surgeons – they always turned to us holding out their ties and we were pleased to oblige. We had several students often coming to learn from our specialists. They were gowned too, of course, but always tied their own sashes. Until one day when only one student came – as usual, he donned his gown and came to me holding out his ties. "Oh no chum," I thought, "you tie your own" and he did!

We were all assembled in the theatre when he turned to me with a lovely smile and flashing dark eyes and requested a stool so that he could sit and observe. Now he really seemed to be going out of his way to annoy me. I'd better deal straightway with this young puppy, and I told him he would find a stool in the next theatre – so he went off and fetched one.

The morning was passing along merrily – all was well. Our surgeon was a very popular older man and we all liked him. Some surgeons had pretty bad tempers, especially one, who always liked the next instrument to be handed to him never deigning to pick it off the trolley even though all were laid out in perfect order, and the instrument must be placed very firmly into his hand, no dithering or he would send it skimming cross the floor.

But this morning we had the man we all liked – he taught us a lot as he went through the operation explaining it to everyone, especially if it was unusual. Such was the next operation. He turned to Sister and requested an instrument which was rarely used – he would need it in about thirty minutes' time – Sister gave me the look and off I went to the next theatre where I knew I'd find the required item.

I went straight to the glass cabinet and was just running my eye along the rows, when I was aware of someone behind me – it was my new friend! He said, "Do you know the instrument Nurse? It's rarely used". Somehow I wasn't too pleased with this intrusion and picked up the instrument, gave him a special look and made my way to the sterilising room without comment.

Always at the end of the list, there was a sense of achievement, and surgeons, Sister and anaesthetists would gather in the office for coffee and biscuits, whilst nurses gathered in their room for refreshment – it was always a relaxed and friendly time.

Unexpectedly a call came from Sister – would I go to her – this sounded ominous – she greeted me with a wide grin and I noticed the others equally tickled. "I'm sorry to interrupt your coffee break, but I would like to introduce you to Mr ...., he is a leading surgeon from a city across the water and has come to observe our theatre techniques". Then we all just burst out laughing – it had certainly been a very good morning for all concerned and one I will always remember.

Strange Ops

One morning I was looking down the list of operations and noticed a name I thought I recognised, but I must be mistaken. This patient had previously been in women's surgical ward and had come in after losing a premature baby – and she was needing treatment. I remembered well how terribly upset she was to have miscarried a longed-for baby. Poor lass, I thought – I knew her age and the chances of becoming pregnant again were slim. So I must be wrong – it couldn't be her coming for a caesarean birth. There were no ultra scanning machines etc and no happy glimpses at tiny hands and toes of the unborn foetus. I just had to find out what was going on. I walked into the anaesthetic room and was greeted with, "Hello nurse, I'm back again". My face must have spoken volumes – she continued. "Yes, it's really me – it was one of twins that I lost – now I'm here for the real thing!"

The patient was right and was delivered of a lovely bonny baby girl. Later I went to the recovery room – what a joyful scene, at last she and her husband had a family.

As I have already said, Christmas on the wards was always lovely and in theatre it was fun too, but different.

Theatre No 2 was taken over, a few decorations were put up, and the operating table had a pretty cloth and tinsel around it. It now formed the buffet.

Someone had found a gramophone and the staff all dressed in fancy garb. I remember that I was a rabbit with lovely bouncy ears.

The day was going well until the phone rang announcing that two victims of a road accident were being admitted for surgery.

So it was off with our fancy dress and on with masks and gowns etc. After a very thorough 'scrub-up', we entered No 1 theatre which of course was awaiting us in its pristine clinical condition.

At the end of the day we had to clear away the party things. My bunny sheet had to go back on my bed, and the cotton wool and bandage ears were popped into the steriliser and would eventually be returned to the dressings box. We had had a very happy Christmas Day.

Theatre Relief

After these three happy months I was due to go back to the wards again, but meanwhile there was a hiccup resulting in a shortage of trained staff for call out at night on theatre duty. That was fine – I promptly volunteered; after all, there was usually little activity during the hours of the night. Ah well, things soon change and it was fairly often after a day of ordinary ward duty that I would be woken by a Night Sister with the call of an operation in approximately twenty minutes – she would have put the necessary instruments into the steriliser to help me. I was happy to get up swiftly, don my uniform and hurry over to the hospital across the lawn and gardens – I loved it.

For small operations the surgeon and anaesthetist were our resident registrars so there was just the three of us – no junior for odd jobs, so I certainly had to see that everything – including any extra for the unexpected – must be prepared. We would put on sterile gowns, masks, caps, boots and gloves after, of course, the ten-minutes 'scrub up'. Night Sister sometimes popped in to see if we needed any help, but she was usually busy, so it was a case of being prepared for anything.

One night had been very busy and Sister called me for the third time. This dressing and undressing lark was becoming tedious, so I decided to wear my pyjamas under my gown – just roll up the legs and no one would have any idea. Now this particular set of nightwear was somewhat garish – brilliant green plant affair material with huge orange poppies – quite eye catching - and so it was that I proceeded into the theatre and carried on as usual. All was going well until I felt that one pyjama leg was slipping slowly down and finally covered my boot! I could do nothing about it - I was all 'scrubbed up' and could not touch anything which was not sterile. I ignored the happening, but the anaesthetist at the head of the patient noticed very promptly and went on to make a general announcement – it was always good to have a distraction during operations in the night, but for some time afterwards I was reminded of this episode!

My very good friend Beau slept in the room next to me and always, whatever time of the night I returned to my bed, would creep in with a welcome warm drink and a biscuit or bun – where did she find them? I never knew how she managed this kindness – she must have had a magic wand or something. She is still a dear friend, but now lives too far away to pop in with sleep inducer.

Ward Rounds

It was now normal night duty on the ward again. I must explain the rules which governed everything: both day and night at the appointed hour – at approximately 10, 2 and 6 o'clock – rounds were carried out. This meant complete inspection, by Matron or any other high ranking Sister, of patients and beds; indeed the whole situation. Nothing was missed, not even an untidy bed or speck of dust.

One rule which was written in stone was that senior nurses, who wore long sleeves after passing certain exams, must always wear their sleeves down – with celluloid-like cuffs on – whenever addressing Matron, or Sisters, or anyone in authority!

This sometimes produced problems – cuffs were often removed in the treatment room or by a patient's bed when attending – well anywhere really, and we all wished that someone would come up with a bright idea for recovery of cuffs. Surely it must be possible to come up with cuffs on invisible retractable thread or the like – but it didn't happen! So, always as Night Sister or Matron was doing the round we walked beside her – giving smoke signals to any available nurse for help. We were most thankful when some dear soul would walk to us and surreptitiously slide cuffs into our waiting hands behind our back.

Occasionally on the men's ward we would hear a patient deciding to give assistance by calling out – "Will someone bring the cuffs please!". Some Sisters smiled; others behaved as if they had forgotten their hearing aid. Yes 'doing the rounds' was always full of unexpected happenings.

This turn of night duty found me as relief nurse; no-one liked being relief, but it was all part of the job.

The usual span of duty was twelve nights on, three nights off. The relief nurses covered these three nights, then moved to the next ward for the next three nights.

We found that the patients always mistrusted the relief – she was never as good as the 'regular' and we really had to try hard to gain their confidence.

It was the first night of a three-night stint on women's surgical. After we had received the report and the day staff had left, we always walked round each bed trying to ascertain what sort of a night lay ahead and meanwhile give any help needed. Finally, I came to a lovely lady in her eighties, just resting on her pillows. I knew from the report that she was very ill and made a mental note to do half-hourly checks.

The hours passed and time for leaving in the morning came – I went over again to dear Margaret. I told her that we were going off duty now. She whispered, "I don't think I'll be here when you come back tonight because I'm very soon going to be with my Lord". I held her hand and stroked her silver hair before leaving her – she was probably right.

But the next night came and I went straight in and peeped to see if Margaret was still with us – yes!! So, as soon as possible I went back to her; she was only semi-conscious and didn't speak; she just lay lifeless and the curtains were pulled around her. My colleague and I popped back every few moments. The rest of the ward was settled for the night and not long before midnight, the junior and I stood together at Margaret's side. Suddenly she sat up – how could she? – her arms outstretched, eyes wide open and a most beautiful smile on that lovely face – then she dropped back to her pillows; she was with her Creator.

A wonderful feeling of calm and peace encompassed that bed, and somehow we were both loathe to leave, and I yearned that one day when my passing comes, it could be as dignified and wonderful as this.

Junior turned and said, "Tonight we have stood on holy ground".

Emergencies

Ah well, no two nights are the same and the next was certainly different.

There was a general feeling of crisis as we reported for duty. I looked into the ward – harassed nurses were scampering around, a trolley was just leaving with a patient for emergency operation, an admission was just arriving and there was a row of beds with new patients all having blood transfusions. The prospects of any quiet nap looked very remote!

I took the report from the worried looking Sister – she was normally ice cool – but not today. There was an illegal abortionist in the area and these women had gone to her for help as they realised they were to have another child to add to their already large brood – now they were fighting for their own lives.

Gradually the day staff went and we were alone. I decided that the situation was desperate and did the unthinkable. No senior nurse must ever leave her ward – ah well, rules are made to be broken – I told the junior I'd be gone for a minute or so; her face said it all.

Rushing to Matron's office, I walked straight in – no knock – just in. It was the Assistant Matron on duty, she looked completely horrified at the intrusion. I demanded some help – at once – no delay – two nurses alone could not cope – I was gone. Within a minute or so I heard familiar footsteps coming towards our ward – it was my pal Beau – she strode in. "I hear you cannot manage the ward without me?" I agreed. A few minutes later another junior appeared, so now we were four and life looked considerably better.

As I said, these women were desperately ill – at death's door – following the shocking treatment and subsequent haemorrhage. The police had been alerted, but the poor souls were too scared to give details. At last we managed to coax one woman to tell us where the house was from which the activities were carried out, but she had no idea of a name. Still there was now enough information for the police to take immediate action and we were thankful to know that the flow of patients coming to our hospital would be halted. The night passed swiftly with trolleys whizzing around. Doctors came in to lend a hand with injections being given to reduce pain and blood loss, drips were constantly renewed, even the Assistant Matron called to ask how things were going. She was very sympathetic and pleased with the amount of order we had achieved, but she didn't offer to stay to help! All the other patients needed attention yet were so considerate especially as they had had little sleep. They all deserved a star.

At last the day staff came along – what a welcome sight – but we still had now to go to the bathroom and sluice through cold water all those sheets that had needed changing. The task seemed endless as we used the little scrubbing brushes and did our best to clean the sheets before packing them into laundry bags. Life is different in the 21st Century! At approximately 11 a.m. it was a case of 'mission complete' and we stumbled off the ward – but first just a look around – it had been an interesting night and also very rewarding. We had not lost one mother and as we left we knew they were all on the long road to recovery.

Children's Ward – Kippers All Round

Children's ward was my next place of sojourn. The ward itself had been rebuilt a few years previously and was very well laid out. The two main wards were in the shape of a semi-circle surrounded by a wide corridor, either side of which were single cubicles, and finally two six-bedded wards. The lower walls were constructed of blue tiles and the upper part was glass, so it was that we could look all around and see most of what was going on … quickly noting problems when needed. All in all, a good design.

It was now some years since they had received quite a few children unexpectedly on this ward, they were evacuated from a bombed hospital in London. Although, of course, the kiddies were discharged when fit enough, that hospital still sent some patients to us and so relieved the beds and space they were trying to use in town. Both patients and relatives seemed to thoroughly enjoy our somewhat rural hospital and facilities.

Our first task in the morning was to prepare and give out breakfast, and make little dishes for our smaller 'fry' and help them to tuck in. To our horror the main kitchen had sent up a supply of kippers as the main part of the meal. Well, I personally had never studied the anatomy of a kipper, but one thing I did know was that they are very well endowed with bones, and bones are not a good ingredient in a small child's diet.

We spent ages filleting the fish, and there were many smiles of amusement from staff and words of encouragement from our ward maid. She was a lively bubbly girl from the Emerald Isle. She kept the ward just spotless and woe betide anyone who dared to walk on her wet floor before she had dried and polished it to perfection. The blue tiles sparkled everywhere and we used to tease her and say that we were going to dispose of the plates and eat directly from the floor.

At last I felt we had done enough – everything possible – and could now give out breakfast and we walked round the corner carrying the food. Wow – suddenly I was sliding along the floor, pieces of kipper going everywhere – walls, ceiling, floor and me. I know that kippers in their former state as herrings swim in the sea – well, these were the flying variety.

The mess was awful; but provoked waves of laughter with some bright soul asking if we had a camera handy. The staff were a grand crowd and helped to recover broken pieces of the large plate and generally clear up everywhere. Even our maid, Maureen, said all was forgiven – she would "soon have things in order again". We went to the main kitchen and left with eggs and quite quickly we were dishing out scrambled eggs, which seemed to be appreciated because little tummies were empty and hungry.

Strange Fruit

It was about this time that we had a visit from chef – a very unlikely happening. He was singing something akin to the Trumpet Voluntary, and he carried in some yellow things – it was the arrival of bananas. We longed to sample one but there were not many and we knew we mustn't – they were only for our children, and very sick patients. So we joyfully introduced them mashed or whole, but the children's faces portrayed what was thought of the new taste, and to our horror they quickly spat out the precious fruit. How could they? We decided that not one scrap should be wasted and we tucked in cheerfully. Bananas tasted wonderful again.

Social Work

As Sister gave the orders for the day she announced that a baby of uncertain age was being admitted that morning. He was a little boy seen by social workers and now coming for general examination and care. She sensed that this might be a case of barrier nursing according to the social worker's report, and I was asked (or rather, told) to be available at the little fellow's arrival.

Mid-morning saw the little deputation enter the office. A very concerned looking social worker accompanied a very poor and pathetic looking mother, scantily dressed and dirty too; her hair needed a thorough wash, she had several front teeth missing and was wearing a completely blank expression, it was impossible to guess her age. They were carrying a dirty bundle of something.

After a brief chat Sister handed the bundle to me – it was a heart stopping moment – little did I guess how much this handful would come to mean to me.

Sister just said, "complete barrier nursing", and indicated the cubicle to which we would go. As soon as mother and social worker left, we began to think how we would cope with this little man. Gently we unravelled him from the filthy blanket and after some discussion with the doctor I was left to begin to clean him up. I undressed him and placed him on a fleece-like sheet. This little soul could only open his eyes halfway as the lids were covered with a sticky goo. His hair was matted so I proceeded with caution and pulled my protective gown around me and pushed every strand of hair securely under my cap. This little fellow was host to head lice and body bugs – he was softly whimpering, not a real cry. At last I'd finally removed everything, all the blankets and clothing, and placed them in the yellow bag for destroying.

It would be impossible to pop him into a soap and water bath. I very carefully began with his eyes, using the finest olive oil and cotton wool and gradually proceeded. He had quite a few nasty little sores. It took ages to attempt to remove the grime from his little head and body, carefully watching for things that jumped.

This was not a job to be completed in one day – it would be repeated several times.

Feeding little Graham was difficult – there was little response, but together we'd make it! So now whilst I was on duty I was to 'special' him and to have no contact with any other patient.

Caring for my little treasure became a happy task – I hardly trusted anyone else to care for him and really wasn't much interested in off duty.

One lovely day he greeted me with a little smile – I hugged him. I was always giving him lots of hugs but now he'd really recognised me – wonderful! Days went by and he was now clean and no longer host to unwanted livestock. His treatment was going well and he was gaining weight at an amazing rate, and so it was that he was pronounced fit enough to join the other little people in the tots ward, and he loved it – now gurgles and smiles were the norm with my dear little lad, but I knew that eventually he would be returned to his mother.

In another cubicle we had a very sick child, a beautiful little boy of two years who was the only child of an older couple. The boy had meningitis – we had no treatment to deal with this.

His parents simply adored him and had moved in with Calum into his cubicle to spend every possible moment with him. Another nurse had the task of specialling him and she grew to love him dearly. We all knew that each day he was weaker and finally he died in his mother's arms. Everyone was terribly upset at this – there were no dry eyes. How different an outcome!

My three months on children's ward were ending. Sister was most considerate and suggested I took my off duty time in the morning when Graham was going home and I was glad. I returned to find an empty cot and a packet of Woodbines as a 'thank you' from his Mum.

One morning when out shopping in the main street of our town, I noticed coming towards me a poor mother pushing a child in a broken pram – I couldn't take it and cowardly crossed the road – meeting my little Graham and his mum was just more than I could bear.

Happy Time

Final examinations were now looming. They were coming nearer by the day and studying was taken very seriously.

A nurse on children's ward doing night duty had gone 'off sick' and so the order came for me to take her place. That I thought was fine. There were always three nurses on children's ward at night, compared to two on everywhere else. But it was good to have three pairs of eyes watching around. Small people change rapidly and babies never call for help – just quietly collapse or something similar, and fade away.

The hours of darkness had gone off well – now it was time to wash or bath everyone. I took two little folk to the bathroom. Johnny was a wee fellow learning to crawl – he had been admitted previously as a very ill child – but now was improving rapidly and was going to be a real charmer. Terry was a poor little scrap, his pale face and large eyes indicated his state – he had kidney failure and was slowly dying – we had no means of lasting help, we could only give him loving attention.

They enjoyed their baths and were now in clean clothes – hair brushed and looking and smelling sweet. I popped Johnny on the floor – he was getting very enthusiastic about this crawling fun and I pointed him in the direction of tots' ward and carried little Terry. Johnny led the way, Terry and I followed and every few minutes we would say "bo" to the little fellow negotiating his way on the floor. Both babies thoroughly enjoyed the "bo" and Terry gave a happy smile, but the effect on Johnny was that each time he just dissolved into giggles, his arms and legs simply collapsed and he lay like a starfish chuckling away and turning his head hoping for another encounter with us. We advanced slowly – I was also, as we all did, casting my eyes through the glass to other places just checking that all was well. Then I noticed another nurse right across the ward giving me frantic signals which I didn't understand – did she need me? No! Then I knew the reason. A voice from behind me said, "Nurse is trying to warn you that I am here!" It was Senior Night Sister come to do her round. I handed over my little charges, pulled on my cuffs and we commenced the 'round' – Sister's eyes did not miss a thing. She spoke kindly to the older children, looked at their story books and played with their toys, and lingered by each cot giving the babies a little tickle under the chin. She would have made a lovely mum.

Sister was a tall impressive woman, very efficient and although appearing to be very severe, could be so kind and helpful in difficult situations as she was a fount of nursing knowledge.

The round was over and we moved towards the double doors – I stepped forward to open them, but she stopped me and turned to ask me why I thought she always left my ward for the last round of the morning – no idea! I was thinking quickly that I had only recently been doing 'relief' so it was different wards every three nights. "I always leave your ward until last because I know that whatever has happened during the night it will be the happiest ward in the hospital". Somehow I managed to breathe a "thank you". Sister gave me a very lovely smile, and opened the door and was gone! I stood still and tried to take in what she had said – I knew that all my life I would never receive a lovelier compliment.

Kitchens

About this time it was considered a great privilege for a nurse to have a few weeks in the kitchen to learn all about diets – this involved studying books and generally preparing dishes. The first morning duty – which seemed to take a long while – was weighing out rations. Larger ones for ward patients, of course, and smaller two ounce rations of butter and a few grains of sugar for staff.

When that was done, I felt rather surplus to requirements and looked around for something to do. So I asked the chef if I could assist him in any task, as the kitchen was always a busy place. The chef was delighted and promptly suggested assembling meat balls. Little did I know what that entailed. He went to the walk-in pantry and emerged staggering under the weight of a large enamel tray loaded with uncooked mince, with the blood all around the tray! I was shown how to roll the mince into the correct size meat ball and he left me to proceed. I spent the rest of my day rolling mince into the required size meat balls!

Strangely enough, it was a long time before I could look into the face of another meat ball. I decided never again to volunteer to assist the chef.

We had no dishwashing machines in those far-off days, it was all hand work.

A lovely lass from Belfast spent her entire day at the deep sink and draining board. She was only young, fifteen or sixteen years old, and had left home looking for work, and this is what she found in England – just washing up – but of course, board and lodging were included. Rosie just kept at it all day, washing up, then drying up when the draining board could hold no more, then off again washing up. As I was looking for something to do, I decided to give Rosie a hand. She was such a merry lass, never complaining, and we got on well, and from then on spare time was always spent at the sink together, laughing as we worked, washing and drying up dishes, pots and pans.

The chef had his kinder side, and always had an excellent supply of birthday cakes. Whenever a patient had such a celebration, he would suitably decorate a cake with name and age.

I was very pleased when my brief spell in the kitchen was over, and I returned to the wards and nursing.

Royalty

During the wartime there were some members of royal families in Europe who had fled from their homeland to find refuge in England, and other friendly countries – and so it was that we had a king come in for treatment at our hospital. He occupied one room on the private patients' block – we rarely saw him – but his wife – a queen of course – had the room next to him and we would quite often see her as she mingled.

One day the rumour was going around that a relative of theirs was coming at 3 p.m. – to visit them both – it was someone we would all like to see. So nurses on night duty and those off duty formed an impromptu guard of honour along the main entrance and the corridor which led off to the private wing.

At 3 p.m. prompt a car drew up and Matron stood on the steps to welcome a princess, tall and elegant.

We were all amazed at how beautiful a woman she was – exquisitely dressed and above all, wearing the most gorgeous perfume which wafted with her as she walked and somehow filled everywhere. We all longed to know just what was this beautiful perfume – but I think that even if we knew, we never could purchase any out of our meagre salary – but it was fun to wish.

Wedding Rings

Beau and I were both planning to marry during the next twelve months and we both longed to get 22 carat gold wedding rings.

Everyone knew that it was almost impossible to obtain such things. All jewellery was very hard to find.

Jewellers' shop windows only had one or two articles on show, maybe a watch or so, but never anything pretty or fancy – the war had not long ended.

One day a jeweller was brought into Beau's ward. He had had a motor bike accident, and it was the usual result – a fracture of the femur. These were always put up on traction and it was a long and protracted time in a hospital bed. Beau decided to take advantage of the situation and enquired about wedding rings. At first the reply was a very definite "no way", but Beau came to know the patient well and she teasingly would threaten all sorts of awful things whilst supporting his leg when his bed was being made or changed. The patient was an older man and really saw the young nurses more like his family. Finally, arrangements were made for Beau and me to visit his shop in the distant future when he was mobile again and back to work.

The appointed day came and we went to see if there was any chance of wedding rings – yes, they were hidden in the back room. We were delighted but the price was a shattering £10 each. Wow! We had not seen a note like that in years – we were earning just over £5 a month – board and lodging paid. Anyhow, we made up our own minds to get the necessary cash, and went back to our rooms to write letters to our future husbands for the money. There were no mobile phones, and phone kiosks were hard to find – so a letter it had to be.

Beau's fiancé was in Dorset in the Army and mine was in the R.A.F. in Stornoway. Eventually, our £10 notes arrived and we went off to buy our wedding rings. We were triumphant, and one day each ring was duly placed, and mine is still on my finger, with a happy memory of a kindly patient.

Rail Crash

One Sunday, fairly early in the morning, we heard that there had been a serious rail crash not far away at Bourne End.

A train had derailed, several carriages had caught fire and rolled down the embankment – there were many injured. The ambulances began arriving – doctors and nurses from other hospitals were brought in, it was all quite chaotic, the corridors and every available space were taken by a trolley. We were a small hospital to deal with this. Our own patients with any degree of fitness were hurriedly sent home and casualties merely suffering from shock were soon treated and sent on their way.

It was a difficult situation and emergency theatres just appeared so that as many travellers as possible could be treated as soon as possible. The smell of burning flesh and material was everywhere and it was difficult to remove the tar-like substance that had formed on people.

Yes, it was hectic and there was never any thought of breaking off for food or a drink. Then suddenly Matron appeared pushing a smaller trolley and on it was milk, sandwiches and glucose. Every worker had to attend her trolley and drink a full glass of milk to which Matron added glucose and there was no mention of not liking milk, then meat sandwiches and finally our name ticked off the list.

So it was that for several days there was very little

order around the hospital, but slowly patients were discharged or transferred to other hospitals. It had certainly been a hectic few days.

Nowadays we hear of violence in our hospitals, but during my nursing days it did not exist. Our very first encounter with anything like that was when a male patient picked up and smashed a glass water jug on the head of a nurse. She was badly concussed and received a large gash on her head – she was off sick for a long time and I'm not sure if she ever nursed again. Some long time after this happened plastic jugs were used, much safer.

Strains

One evening as we walked onto the ward to commence night duty we just did our usual "Good evening everyone" – and we were met by a loud reply, "Thank goodness you are here – I'm very ill and no one will listen!" Recognition was immediate; it was Mrs Norton.

Now, Mrs Norton was a regular hospital bird, always returning to roost at odd intervals. She had had various illnesses and a selection of fractures! She was also a rather large lady. Earlier in the day Mrs Norton had been admitted with a fractured ankle – the necessary treatment had been given and she was now in plaster from toes to knee and had been placed with leg support under a cage. Plaster took quite a long while to dry in the 1940s and we needed to keep bed covers off the leg. Mrs Norton was always in a hurry for attention and was complaining of severe pain – we assured her we would be along shortly. As I arrived at her bed, I automatically placed my fingers over her pulse – my goodness! It was racing. So drawing the curtains around her bed, I told her I'd like to look at her abdomen. I was not being entirely honest – gazing at Mrs Norton's tummy was like looking at a replica of the Rock of Gibraltar. Finding the site of her appendix, which was my aim, would not be easy, but fortunately the spot was quickly found with our patient just about hitting the ceiling. Yes – this time it was for real, and arrangements were made for surgery that night. It was decided to move our patient on her bed to theatre as this would lessen the strain on staff backs.

In the small hours Mrs Norton returned to the ward, barely conscious. We needed to lift her as high as possible into the sitting position so as to assist drainage and avoid complication.

Well, my colleague and I tried hard with little success, but a doctor from theatre had already foreseen this slight hiccup and came to help – but no way. We rang for a porter, a burly fellow, and so with much huffing and puffing on everyone's part, including the patient, whose puffs were mixed with moans, we achieved our objective.

The next thing was to insert the donkey under her knees as soon as possible. Now, the donkey was not of the four-footed variety, it was an elongated pillow type thing with ties at either side – firmly placed under the knees – ties tucked in under the mattress at both sides, and so the patient was held in the sitting position.

The donkey is no longer in use as there were fears that it could cause deep vein thrombosis, but personally I never encountered a case.

Mrs Norton progressed well and was discharged to prepare for her next visit to hospital.

Visiting time in those days was a highly organised affair. The hours were strictly adhered to; anyone staying after the 'end of visiting' bell was sounded found themselves facing Sister or Staff Nurse who gave a few words.

Only two visitors per bed at any time were allowed and no-one ever sat on the bed.

Transferring of bugs was just not allowed – either those of infection or any of the hopping species.

Chapter Four

Final Exams

So the days sped by and the time for the written exams and the orals had nearly arrived.

Testing Times

There were at this time many cases of poliomyelitis – or infantile paralysis – throughout the country, little was really known about it and there was much concern. One doctor who used to visit our hospital to lecture realised the need for training of staff as to this disease and so gave a course of lectures; he was positive that a question on this subject would be on our exam papers.

We studied hard and I was very confident that I knew everything about the effect of polio on nerves and muscles – and the way of treatment – or as much as was then known. That treatment sometimes necessitated a stay in an iron lung – now that was a contraption of frightening proportions. When switched on, it strongly assisted with breathing. A volunteer was requested to show just how efficient it was. Our one and only male nurse volunteered – all very macho! Well, after a very short time he had to be released as he had gone a dreadful colour and was in need of first aid. At least we had added to our learning.

On the appointed day we entered the large hall and went to our desks – all well spaced out, so we sat down and looked at the question papers. I read through and through but there was absolutely nothing about polio – to think of all my knowledge being wasted. I made a mental note of what I would say at my next encounter with the knowledgeable young doctor. Ah well, there were plenty of other demanding questions and I commenced the task in hand. After several hours we had a break and then more papers to be answered.

Somehow the day went by and I remember returning to my own hospital and finally my room, by which time I was feeling pretty exhausted. Some girls were going to look up their text books to see what they had missed – I didn't pursue this fruitless road. What is done is done!

Orals

In a few days it was time for the oral examinations. There would be four interviews. The first one was surgical – that should be fine – the call came for me to enter the 'lions' den'. At the desk sat a very foreboding middle-aged man. "Morning," he bellowed at me. "Sit down". Well, I was now very apprehensive and just sat on the edge of the chair. Again the voice – "I said sit down". I took this to mean that I must sit further back in the chair. We proceeded. He threw a question at me, "Hearts or hernias, which shall we talk about?" I quickly answered "hearts". I knew quite a lot about these but not hernias – I never did like hernias. "Right!" was his next statement, "We'll talk about hernias". This was a bad start and so it went on with me sinking further into the mire with every question. I couldn't remember a thing properly – he seemed to have cast a spell or something over me. At last he told me to "go". I retreated like a jelly fish and knew that he must have written a large 'failure'. Did the Human Rights Committee know about this man?

I sank into the chair which some kindly person had placed outside and awaited the next call. Both the second and third interviewers were quite normal people and I was able to know the answers. The final interrogation was with a motherly soul and the answers flowed freely. The minutes went quickly by and at the end she said, "Well done" and wished me luck.

We had come to the end of examinations; now we wondered what our ward reports would contain – it could make a lot of difference.

Results

It's strange how time seems to go by very slowly when we are anxiously waiting for something and so it was that I tried hard to keep extra busy as I awaited the morning when the results would be made known.

There were three of us on one ward and we all in the same state – waiting.

When the day dawned, we knew that we must wait until coffee break and receive the results over in the Home - that was always the last port of call for the porter carrying the post.

Well, one of our threesome decided that things would be different and she went to the Main Hall and watched the porter's lodge. As soon as the porter went off on some other errand she dived in and went through the postbag until she found our three envelopes – how dare she? Still, we gave her a sincere welcome when she arrived back on the ward as we waited with bated breath.

One of the nurses was a much older girl – quite old, all of thirty years! She opened her envelope and burst into tears – happy tears? No – she had failed. With trembling hands I opened mine – I still have the letter. I read 'We have much pleasure……' – wonderful! – I'd come through – I'd won through – I was a State Registered Nurse!

The road on which I had travelled to reach my goal had sometimes been a little rough, but mostly smooth, and I thoroughly enjoyed it all. I met some lovely people and made good friends ……..

I would gladly walk this road again.

Contract of Service

WEST HERTS HOSPITAL,
HEMEL HEMPSTEAD.

CONDITIONS OF SERVICE

AND

AGREEMENT FOR THE ENGAGEMENT

OF STUDENT NURSES.

WEST HERTS HOSPITAL,
HEMEL HEMPSTEAD.

The West Herts Hospital is an old established hospital having occupied a previous site before the present one. Much of the present building is new, and contains 173 in-patient beds. There are male and female medical and surgical wards, a children's ward, a private block, a maternity unit and an Out-Patients Department.

The twin operating theatres are among the most up to date in the country, and the new x-Ray department is fitted with modern equipment. The children's ward is a delightful block opened in 1940 and has 30 cots. Everything possible was done when planning the building to provide an efficient unit of modern design.

The Hospital's Honorary Medical Staff includes Consultants from London hospitals, and thousands of in and out-patients receive treatment every year.

Nurses are coached throughout their training by a qualified resident Sister Tutor; lectures are given by her and by members of the honorary medical staff. During training visits of interest are arranged to neighbouring factories, water works, ventilation plants, etc.

The welfare of the nurses is supervised by a Home Sister. The nurse's health is watched carefully during her training and should a nurse be ill she receives full medical attention free of charge.

The hospital is pleasantly situated ; country and town being easily accessible. Student Nurses are allowed to bring bicycles and they spend many happy hours exploring the delightful county of Hertford. For those who prefer the town there is a good bus and train service into London.

Recreation facilities provided include a hard tennis court, table tennis, radiogram and an up-to-date library of fiction and nursing text books. The grounds of the hospital are pleasant and the nurses' home has a flat roof for sunbathing. There is a visitors room in the home where nurses may entertain their visitors when off duty.

There is a charming little Chapel in the hospital. For those who wish to attend there are "prayers" each evening at 8.30 and on Sundays the hospital Chaplain conducts a short service at 5.30 p.m. which convalescent patients may also attend. An early morning Communion service is held twice a month.

CONDITIONS OF SERVICE FOR STUDENT NURSES

who are candidates for admission to the General Part of the State Register of Nurses

Conditions of Acceptance

1. Every candidate is asked to complete and return the application form to the matron, who will make an appointment to give the candidate a personal interview at the hospital.
2. Candidates should be over the age of 17½ years.
3. Before being accepted every candidate is required to furnish an official copy of her birth certificate and to satisfy the matron as to her health by certificates on the prescribed forms.
4. Candidates are also required to undergo a medical examination at the hospital.

Preliminary Training School

5. Before going on the wards candidates will be required to enter the Preliminary Training School for a short course of instruction. During such training candidates will be paid at the rate of £40 per annum and will be provided with board, lodging and laundry, as well as with the official indoor uniform prescribed by the regulations in force.

Trial Period

6. On completion of the Preliminary Training School course approved candidates will be admitted to the hospital as Student Nurses for a trial period of twelve weeks. During this period their services may be terminated if they are found unsuitable in any respect, or the candidate, if she finds practical hospital work uncongenial, may leave at her own request upon giving written notice to the matron.

Conditions on Engagement

7. Student nurses are accepted for training by the Governing Body upon the recommendation of the matron and must have successfully completed the trial period. They are then required to sign an agreement by which they are received as Student Nurses in training for the State Registration examinations. The agreement will cover a period of four years' training, which includes the Preliminary Training School course and the trial period above referred to.

Hospital Training and Examinations

8. Student nurses are given theoretical and practical training in accordance with the syllabus laid down by the General Nursing Council for England and Wales, being instructed by the sister tutor and sisters, and by the medical and surgical staff appointed by the hospital for the purpose.
9. Every student nurse will have been prepared for and will be required to have entered for the Preliminary State Examination Parts I. and II. by the end of her first year of training, or at the examination next following. In the event of a student nurse failing to pass the Preliminary State Examination at the second attempt the Governing Body may terminate her engagement.
10. After passing the Preliminary State Examination every student nurse is required to take the Final State Examination, the hospital undertaking to provide the necessary facilities for her preparation before the completion of three years of her training. She is also required to take the internal examinations, conducted at the hospital by its own examiners.
11. Every student nurse who completes her full period of training to the satisfaction of the Governing Body, has passed the State Examination and has passed the internal examinations, if any, will be awarded a certificate signed by the chairman or vice-chairman of the Governing Body, appropriate members of the medical and surgical staff and the matron of the hospital.

Conditions of Service

12. Student nurses receive free board and lodging and live in the nurses' home or in other provided accommodation. Indoor uniform and laundry are provided. Student nurses are medically examined at regular intervals.

3

Salary is paid monthly in arrear, beginning from the date of the commencement of training (including any period in the Preliminary Training School) on the following scales :—

	Salary	Value of Emoluments	Total Value of Salary and Emoluments
1st year	£40 p.a.		£115 p.a.
2nd year	£45 p.a.		£120 p.a.
3rd year	£50 p.a.	£75 p.a.	£125 p.a.
4th year (until State Registered)	£60 p.a.		£135 p.a.
4th year (after State Registered)	£70 p.a.		£145 p.a.

13. Student nurses are required to participate in the Federated Superannuation Scheme for Nurses and Hospital Officers (Contributory) on completion of one year's training. [Particulars of the scheme may be obtained on application to the hospital].

14. Student nurses are under the authority of the matron and are required to obey the instructions of their superior officers and, in professional matters, of the medical staff. They work in the wards and departments of the hospital as allocated by the matron and are required to undertake night duty for a period normally not exceeding four months at a time.

15. Student nurses' specified hours of duty, off duty times and annual leave are adhered to as closely as possible but are subject to the exigencies of the hospital's service.

16. Student nurses are normally on duty for an average of 96 hours per fortnight, exclusive of meals and inclusive of compulsory lectures.

17. The prescribed periods of daily and weekly off duty and annual leave are as follows :—

    3 to 4 hours off duty daily.
    1 day off per week.
    4 weeks' annual leave (in one or more parts).

During annual leave student nurses will receive in addition to their salary an allowance of 15/- per week.

18. On production of a medical certificate sick leave with pay, reduced by an amount equivalent to the statutory benefit by which a Student Nurse may become entitled under the National Health Insurance Acts, will be granted up to the following periods :—

During the first year	1 month's full pay and (after 4 months' service) two months' half pay.
During the second year	2 months' full pay and 2 months' half pay.
During the third year and subsequent years	3 months' full pay and 3 months' half pay.

If the student nurse is not being provided by the hospital with in-patient treatment she will receive during the periods of sick leave, in lieu of board and residence, an allowance of 15/- per week, while on full pay, and 7/6 per week, while on half pay."

19. If the student nurse is unable to resume her duties at the end of the appropriate prescribed periods her engagement will thereupon be deemed to be automatically terminated without notice. The Governing Body may at its discretion, extend the period of sick leave (with or without pay). Any such discretionary payment by the hospital to the nurse will not create a fresh agreement of employment and training, and may be discontinued at any time without liability on the part of the hospital to give notice.

20. Any time lost beyond seven days a year cannot be counted in the period of training and must be made up before the four years can be considered complete.

---

* A student nurse who is exempted from Health Insurance on the ground of assured private income shall pay to the hospital the amount of sickness benefit to which she would have been entitled if she had been insured.

21. If a student nurse becomes entitled to any allowance under the Workmen's Compensation Acts, she shall, while remaining in residence, make such payment to the hospital as the Governing Body shall decide.

22. A student nurse wishing to marry is required to give the hospital one month's notice of her intention and on her marriage her contract as a student nurse will thereby be terminated without prejudice to the renewal of her contract being considered by the Governing Body.

23. Any student nurse leaving the service of the hospital voluntarily and without express permission may be required to pay a forfeit of—

If in the first year of training	£6
If in the second year of training	£7
If in the third year of training	£8
If in the fourth year of training	£10

24. The matron may suspend a student nurse from duty at any time during her training, reporting the same to the Governing Body immediately, and the Governing Body may terminate the contract of any student nurse at any time without notice for neglect of duty, disobedience, misconduct or other sufficient cause.

Note to Hospital—The form should be signed by both parties in duplicate, the original being retained by Hospital, the duplicate by the Nurse.

FORM 1. (Applicable where the Student Nurse is 21 years of age or more).

FORM OF AGREEMENT FOR ENGAGEMENT OF STUDENT NURSE

AN AGREEMENT made the .... day of 19   BETWEEN

the WEST HERTS HOSPITAL (hereinafter called the Hospital) of the one part and.................................

....of... (hereinafter called the student nurse) of the other part.

WHEREBY IT IS AGREED AS FOLLOWS :—

1. The Hospital agrees to engage the student nurse as from the.................. day of 19   on the terms and conditions set out in the Conditions of Service for Student Nurses printed on the back of this agreement and to provide her with the necessary training for the State Examinations and for the Hospital Certificate.

2. The student nurse agrees to serve the Hospital as a student nurse for the period of .... years from the.........................day of 19   and to conform to the said Conditions of Service and to the regulations of the Hospital from time to time in force relating to student nurses as though these conditions and regulations formed part of this agreement.

3. If before the expiration of the said period the student nurse leaves the service of the Hospital voluntarily and without the express permission of the Hospital, she will pay to the Hospital the sum of £6 if she leaves in the first year of her service, £7 if in the second year, £8 if in the third year, £10 if in the fourth year, such sum to be by way of liquidated damages and recoverable from her as a debt due to the Hospital.

AS WITNESS our hands the day and year first above written.

....*(Student Nurse)*.

....*(Matron)*.
Matron of the Hospital, for and on behalf of the Hospital

6

Note to Hospital—The form should be signed by both parties in duplicate, the original being retained by Hospital, the duplicate by the Nurse.

FORM 2. (Applicable where the Student Nurse is under 21 years of age).

FORM OF AGREEMENT FOR ENGAGEMENT OF STUDENT NURSE

AN AGREEMENT made the .... day of .... 19 BETWEEN the WEST HERTS HOSPITAL (hereinafter called the Hospital) of the one part and................................ ....of.. (hereinafter called the student nurse) of the second part, and..of..parent (or guardian) of the student nurse of the third part

WHEREBY IT IS AGREED AS FOLLOWS :—

1. The Hospital agrees to engage the student nurse as from the.................. day of 19   on the terms and conditions set out in the Conditions of Service for Student Nurses printed on the back of this agreement and to provide her with the necessary training for the State Examinations and for the Hospital Certificate.

2. The student nurse agrees to serve the Hospital as a student nurse for the period of four years from the.........................day of 19   and to conform to the said Conditions of Service and to the regulations of the Hospital from time to time in force relating to student nurses as though these conditions and regulations formed part of this agreement.

3. If before the expiration of the said period the student nurse leaves the service of the Hospital voluntarily and without the express permission of the Hospital, she will pay to the Hospital the sum of £6 if she leaves in the first year of her service, £7 if in the second year, £8 if in the third year, £10 if in the fourth year, such sum to be by way of liquidated damages and recoverable from her as a debt due to the Hospital.

4. In consideration of the Hospital engaging the student nurse as hereinbefore provided the said .... guarantees the payment by the student nurse of any sum or sums payable by her by virtue of this agreement.

AS WITNESS our hands the day and year first above written.

....(*Student Nurse*).

....(*Matron*).
Matron of the Hospital, for and on behalf of the Hospital.

....(*Parent or Guardian*).

Lightning Source UK Ltd.
Milton Keynes UK
05 January 2011

165221UK00001B/16/P